Kathi's an unmatched therapist, ph
with a healing soul and a compassi
copy of

John Williams, Composer/Conductor, Boston Pops, Boston Symphony Orchestra

The Fairbend Method to Achieve Sound Posture and Better Mood

STAND UP TO DEPRESSION

How To Activate THE BODY MIND MIRACLE And Defeat Depression

Includes Exercises with Diagrams and Written Descriptions

Kathi Fairbend, MS RPT

Foreword by Keith Ablow, MD

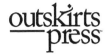

STAND UP TO DEPRESSION
How To Activate THE BODY MIND MIRACLE And Defeat Depression
All Rights Reserved.
Copyright © 2020 Kathi Fairbend, MS RPT
v4.0

The opinions expressed in this manuscript are solely the opinions of the author and do not represent the opinions or thoughts of the publisher. The author has represented and warranted full ownership and/or legal right to publish all the materials in this book.

This book may not be reproduced, transmitted, or stored in whole or in part by any means, including graphic, electronic, or mechanical without the express written consent of the publisher except in the case of brief quotations embodied in critical articles and reviews.

Outskirts Press, Inc.
http://www.outskirtspress.com

ISBN: 978-1-9772-1760-8

Library of Congress Control Number: 2019912830

Cover Photo © 2020 www.gettyimages.com. All rights reserved - used with permission.

Outskirts Press and the "OP" logo are trademarks belonging to Outskirts Press, Inc.

PRINTED IN THE UNITED STATES OF AMERICA

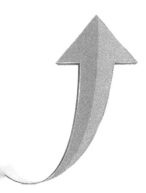

Foreword

So much has been written about the mind-body connection—and rightfully so. It now seems obvious that our psychological state affects the function not only of the central nervous system, but the heart and every organ in the body. Diseases from cancer to multiple sclerosis to hypertension, and everything in between, demonstrate undeniable links to depression, emotional trauma and unresolved, underlying anger.

We are lucky to have recognized the ways that yoga can stave off dementia and the ways that meditation can increase longevity.

Too little, however, has been written about the mirror image of the mind-body connection—*the body-mind connection*. Yet we do know that correcting bodily abnormalities can correct emotional ones. Certainly, exercise can improve mood, but that isn't half the story. We are learning incredible ways in which one's psychological equilibrium can be optimized by optimizing one's physical equilibrium.

Simply put, developing physical balance is key to developing emotional balance. This is not theory, anymore; it is fact. One example: Botox, which prevents the brow from furrowing when we worry, also seems to short-circuit worry itself. Botox will soon be approved to treat major depression. When we relax the muscles that contract too powerfully when we are over-wrought, the mind seems to relax, too.

Another example: Probiotics that alter bacterial colonization of the gut can insulate the mind from profound highs and lows of mood.

These examples are just the beginning. Our bodily state influences our mental state in myriad ways. And it is to this growing field of knowledge that physical therapist Kathi Fairbend, MS, RPT adds her crucial contribution. *Stand Up to Depression* makes the simple, elegant and powerful point that correcting one's posture can literally pave the way to elevating one's mood. As Fairbend makes plain, if you teach yourself to stand up like a person who isn't depressed, you will be in a better position (quite literally) to *become* a person who isn't depressed.

Think about it: If using Botox to block the contractions of a few muscles in one's forehead can treat depression, imagine what can happen when (with the help of Ms. Fairbend's book) you learn to stand up to depression, stop slouching, walk confidently and plant your feet firmly on the ground. Dozens of your muscles will resonate with your intention to stand up straight in life, shoulder your troubles and refuse the negative feedback that comes from inadvertently bending an ankle or buckling a knee, with every step you take.

Depression is insidious. It hobbles its victims mentally, but also physically. Reverse the physical decline, and it helps to reverse the mental decline.

It has been my great honor to consult to Ms. Fairbend as she wrote her groundbreaking book. I have had a front row seat to the birth of a new specialty of physical therapy—*physical therapy for the mind*. And I can envision a time when, with Kathi's help, thousands of physical therapists will treat hundreds of thousands of patients who come to them not only for help with joints and muscles and bones, but for help with depression and anxiety.

For now, that help can come directly from this book. *Stand Up to Depression* stands alone as the way that people around America and around the world can tap into the brilliance of (as I see it) America's leading physical therapist, a woman whose entire life's work makes her uniquely qualified to take her readers on a bold new path of healing.

Keith Ablow, MD

Table of Contents

Part 1: The Invisible/Visible Solution

Profile of Depression 3

The Body Mind Miracle 17

Spectrum of Depression 27

Secondary Health Problems 36

**Part 2: Learning The Fairbend Method
to *Stand up to Depression***

Ergonomic Health and Productivity in the Workplace are
        Influenced by Posture and Mood 47

Developing Individualized Exercise Programs 57

Exercise Instructions to Improve Posture and
        Mood and *Stand Up to Depression* 64

Maintaining Sound Posture to *Stand Up to Depression* 87

Afterword: Believing in Simplicity...90

About the Author..91

Acknowledgements 94

Physical Therapy for The Mind...96

Part 1:
The Invisible/ Visible Solution

1

Profile of Depression

Mood affects posture, and posture affects mood. It's a simple equation. But people have difficulty making the connection—and believing it. Even "Conrad," an active, retired astronomy professor quite capable of articulating sophisticated beliefs about life on other planets, wasn't quite sure his muscles and joints could be affecting his mood when I began working with him.

You might think a man like Conrad, while taking a walk, would be gazing at the stars or pondering the endless dimensions of outer space. If you'd seen him walking in your neighborhood, however, you'd probably have thought he'd been condemned to the guillotine. He looked down at his feet, studying the sidewalk. His shoulders were rounded, his pants dragged, and, much to his dismay, his belly stuck out, even though he wasn't overweight. Meanwhile, he worried incessantly about his health, and, in his words, "what might happen." He called his physician with endless questions about a myriad of diseases and made numerous unnecessary trips to the emergency room with complaints of chest pain, shortness of breath and abdominal pain. Tests always proved negative: His health was excellent for an active 69-year-old man.

Conrad's body told the real story of what afflicted him—depression. That's what had him hunched over, not looking forward (physically or emotionally), anymore.

"Should I lose a few pounds?" he repeatedly asked me.

"No, Conrad," I told him. "You should speak to your physician, or possibly a psychiatrist, about depression."

"You think I'm depressed? My friends worry about that."

"I do, Conrad. And you know what, you *look* depressed. Your body shows it. And you do have to talk to someone about getting help. But we can fight the depression, too."

"How?" he asked.

"By standing up to it—literally," I said.

After four months working with Conrad, teaching him techniques to improve his posture and the way he walked (his gait), Conrad proudly asked me to assess his body position and walking speed. He reported that one of his neighbors had complimented his powerful stride. Here's the really wonderful part, though: His mood was better. He was more optimistic. He felt stronger. And he credited the changes in his outlook both to achieving the "stance," physically, of a person without depression, as well as to thinking about moving forward in life with his new psychologist.

That shouldn't surprise anyone. Think of the word *outlook*. It's pretty tough to look forward in life, if you're hunched over.

Magnitude of Depression

Depression is the leading cause of disability worldwide. The World Health Organization (WHO) states that, globally, more than 300 million people of all ages suffer from the insidious malady. At its worst, it can lead to suicide, despite the availability of effective treatments. And there *are* very effective treatments. But one strategy—literally, *standing up to depression*—has been ignored. No more.

I am not saying that those suffering with depression should reject psychotherapy or medications or wonderful new treatments like ketamine or dTMS (deep transcranial magnetic stimulation). I am saying that all those treatments target the brain and mind, leaving aside the way that the body—literally, its muscles and joints—powerfully influences the mind.

The National Institutes of Health (NIH) reported in 2016 that an estimated 16.2 million adults had suffered one major depressive episode in that year. That represents 6.7 percent of the adult population.

With the vast number of afflicted people, one would think that experts would have noted that major depression doesn't just attack mood, energy, self-esteem, sleep, appetite and concentration. It affects the body—visibly and dramatically. This is true whether the depressed person is sitting, standing or walking.

Later in this book, I will explain how The Fairbend Method will help you stand up to depression by disrupting poor posture and improving body movement. But, first, let's review some of the physical signs of depression that a person with depression can (unconsciously) display while sitting, standing or walking.

The depressed *sitting* posture has many of the following characteristics:

- Head forward in front of the shoulders.

- Back curled.

- Knees folded, with feet up on the chair, often twisted to one side, apparently to take up very little space.

- Eyes staring toward the ground, as though shutting down and shutting out the world.

I have frequently seen patients in my waiting room, sitting with their heads in their hands, elbows on their knees. Sometimes, their heads are literally in their open palms, which are down on their thighs. And they don't realize that repeatedly assuming this posture—and others like it—gives their minds the message that they can't face the day.

Most common *standing* posture of the depressed patient:

- Head forward and down, well in front of the shoulders.

- Shoulders rounded, so that there is no "room" for the head to be lifted.

- Forward curvature of the upper back, with resulting forward curvature of spine (kyphosis).

- Arms hanging well ahead of the shoulders rather than at the side (picture a chimp).

- Protruding abdomen from being pushed out by the "C" shape of the spine.

As with sitting, when the head is pulled forward it twists the spine and causes the chest to collapse. This standing posture also causes the belly to protrude, which is what the depressed person usually notices.

If you're depressed, and all this sounds familiar, take heart. Standing up to depression can be a critical component in your healing strategy.

If you're a relative or friend of a depressed person, please notice these features of his or her posture. Kindly commenting on what you've observed and suggesting that correcting their posture, through the methods described in this book, can be one of the keys to overcoming depression, would be a wonderful gift to give that person. Of course, since this method is not a "cure all," other resources (such as those of a psychiatrist) will also likely be essential.

The *gait or walking* pattern in a depressed person:

- Slow, inefficient and demonstrates poor balance.

- Feet dragging.

- Noticeable lack of endurance.

- Head and eyes looking at ground.

- The gait is frequently determined by the standing position, as described above. This is because the change in the alignment/position of the pelvis (while standing) causes one's body weight to be thrown forward. The feet have to try to hold the whole body steady, even though the body is a series of curves, instead of a straight line. This negatively impacts balance, while also creating strain on the low back.

These harmful postures must be addressed or they will affect and prolong depressed mood, lack of energy, impaired breathing, decreased productivity and poor overall health. Standing, sitting and walking in these "depressed" ways certainly impacts self-esteem, negatively. The Fairbend Method targets these bodily signs of depression and reverses them, which allows the body to function in synchrony and the mind to take notice.

And, please remember, unconscious bad habits when sitting and standing are not only part of the portrait of depression, but may not be noticed by the depressed person him or herself. So, it may fall on families and colleagues to take note of them and urge the individual to address them.

The good news is that depression responds so well to treatment. In addition to psychotherapy and medications, strides in neuroscience have led to the development of new treatments such as deep transcranial magnetic stimulation (dTMS) and the use of ketamine. Both these new treatments are approved by the FDA. Exercise is also essential in regaining self-esteem, health and overall wellbeing. The point is that a comprehensive approach is the key. Standing up to depression ought to be part of that comprehensive approach.

Why Stand Up to Depression

In a career spanning decades, I have been astounded to see so many cases of depression intertwined with orthopedic problems, including poor posture. Severe or untreated scoliosis (an "S" type curvature of the spine, from side to side) or kyphosis (an exaggerated forward curvature of the spine) are frequently seen in adolescents and can be the result of untreated osteoporosis in older adults. Both scoliosis and kyphosis, can be discouraging, disfiguring and painful. They can limit a person's cherished independence. And they can pave the way for depression to take hold.

"Sally" had to stop driving at the age of 56 after an auto accident. The collision occurred because her severe scoliosis eventually altered the position of her head, tilting it to one side, resulting in compromised vision and depth perception. Since she had to give up driving after her accident, which caused some social isolation, Sally suffered a significant depressive episode.

Depression may also be triggered in a child with severe scoliosis who must wear a brace throughout the middle school years. Doctors generally know that untreated scoliosis potentially sets the stage for chronic pain and even damage to internal organs, but fewer focus on the damage to self-esteem that the condition can cause. Back braces themselves can make young people feel damaged and different from their classmates.

Scoliosis is a far cry from the conditions experienced by Conrad. His depression caused his problems with muscles, joints and posture. In the case of scoliosis in a young person, it is far more likely that the physical problem precedes the emotional fallout. Yet both scenarios can be effectively treated with *The Fairbend Method.* Why? Because they share a common denominator: Mood affects posture, and posture affects mood.

It's a complex interplay. Fitness fanatics are another example of a group who can be afflicted by poor posture and, then, by depression. Why? Too often their exercise regimes become unhealthy obsessions that rule their lives. When sidelined by an injury, members of this group—much like a professional skier who is involved in a skiing accident—can descend into major depressive episodes.

Some fitness devotees are prisoners of a vicious cycle. They take up exercise to combat blue or dark moods. When they cycle, lift weights or become marathon runners, endorphins (hormones) in the brain and nervous system are released, reducing their sense of pain. It's a wonderful, natural way to improve one's perception of life—until an injury intercedes and makes exercising impossible. Then, the brain ends up starved for those extra endorphins.

When I met "Kara" for the first time she offered her own diagnosis. "I have sciatic nerve problems. My doctor told me I overused my hip muscles and irritated or compressed the nerve. He said it's called piriformis syndrome. I've had it in the past, but now the muscle spasms in my back, buttock area and leg are constant," she said.

As we talked, I assessed her physical symptoms. She presented with very rounded shoulders. Her head and neck were thrust forward. Kyphosis (the outward curve of the upper back, discussed above) was obvious. Her belly protruded.

Does all this sound familiar? Clearly, this type of posture is not what you might expect of an athlete, but it is common among depressed people.

Depressed mood and low self-esteem may be *invisible*, but posture is *visible* and very revealing about mental health.

"I haven't been able to work out or run for ten days," Kara said with no small amount of anguish and frustration.

"On a scale of zero to ten, how would you rate your pain?"

"Ten!"

"Okay. Do you remember when the spasms and pain began?" These mishaps can occur even after chores we consider normal or hum-drum.

"Well, I carried two paddle boards up some stairs."

"From your basement or—?"

"No. We were at the beach."

"Ah. So, you had to climb those stairs twice and—"

"No," she scoffed. "I carried them both at the same time. I mean, heck, it was a 75-step climb, after walking in the sand. I didn't want to do that twice."

Kara was accustomed to running 30 to 40 miles a week and either biking 20 miles a day or using an elliptical training machine for an hour a day. Her goal was to get in tip-top shape over a 4-month period, so that she could run a marathon to celebrate her 60th birthday. In the previous 6 to 7 months, she had worked with 12 different trainers and performed 8 different fitness routines.

The intensity of Kara's workout history and mind-set was a red flag. One the toughest aspects of my work is to speak truth to power by explaining to patients with exercise addictions that their excessive exercise is causing them to injure their bodies. They may well have begun as a way to cope with underlying problems of mood.

My first goal was to ease Kara's painful cycle of muscle spasms so that the tissue could rest and heal. My suggestion to Kara was that she start with a conservative 10-day physical therapy routine. After sharing the details, it was time for me to lower the boom. "Kara," I told her, "this means you cannot work out or run until you are pain free, and I suggest that you take some anti-inflammatory medications."

"Uh-uh. No drugs."

It was her right to decline medications, of course. "Okay, then it's going to be even more important to ice the area four times daily and rest for up to five hours each day."

"I can't do *anything*?" she asked.

"Sure. You can walk several times a day, outside, for 10 to 15 minutes," I suggested, hoping this would be enough to appease her zeal for exercise. Then I added three gentle stretches, which she was instructed to do three or four times per day.

"Why the stretches?"

"They'll help break up the muscle spasms. These are all simple, positive actions that will reduce your pain."

Withdrawal from any addiction is difficult. Kara's dependency on physical exertion was as strong as any I'd seen. She teared up, but said she would go forward with the plan.

Days later, on a follow-up visit, Kara was accompanied by "Vince," her husband. She rated her pain at 7, a significant drop since her first visit, but Vince had other things on his mind.

"I have connections in the medical community," Vince said. "I can get any surgeon you think is suitable." This was not a direction I was ready to recommend, but he persisted. "Kara feels like her life has ended. She wants us to sell the house and move into a condo. I'm not ready for that. *We're* not ready. We've got to *do* something."

Profile of Depression

The need to act in a time of crisis is understandable. Yet if the affliction—depression—remains invisible, the action taken may miss the mark.

Instead of encouraging Vince to find a surgeon, I suggested that he speak with a brilliant orthopedic surgeon with an engineering background, who had himself stopped performing surgery to focus on providing consultations. I knew they would receive a thorough evaluation, a professional opinion and, if needed, a recommendation for an excellent surgeon. Thankfully, both Kara and Vince agreed to the consultation.

Fortunately, Kara's depression improved when an MRI revealed a cyst resting near her sciatic nerve. The cyst was the result of overusing muscles, causing trauma to soft tissues in that area. In Kara's case, the cyst was pressing on the sciatic nerve. It was not a dangerous scenario and, with conservative treatment to eliminate excessive movement, the cyst dissolved, and her pain disappeared.

The MRI that revealed Kara's cyst provided me with an opportunity to implement a conservative physical therapy program that included tissue healing, stretching and strengthening exercises, plus major improvements to her body mechanics and the ergonomics in her home environment. I was very careful to include many elements of The Fairbend Method, because I knew that depression had been part of the fuel for Kara's extreme exercise regimen. And standing up to that depression (literally, of course) could be one way to combat it.

Kara became pain free without the need for surgery. Her mood improved as her posture improved. Vince did not sell the farm and retire from life as he had known it.

Is it really so simple? Yes, in most cases, it is simple. The body affects the mind, and the mind affects the body. Pay attention to both, and better results are likely.

How the Mind Influences Body Movement

The problem is awareness: invisible versus visible. Blindness versus perception. Many people would choose to try to "fix" pain with surgical tools, rather than admit to a deeper problem. That's why I consider my work with athletes to be "physical therapy for the mind," not sports medicine or "body work." Physical symptoms won't necessarily improve if the individual in pain is unwilling to look within.

For a moment, let's forget about the physical pain that led to Kara's depression. It turned out there were other factors impacting her emotional state, including problems in her marriage. These problems had been fueling a brewing depression. And that's what depression is often like—an off-shore storm that is ignored, until it finally hits land and causes immeasurable collateral damage (in her case to muscles and nerves).

Even as she recovered, Kara was unwilling to see the connection between mind and body. She told her adult son that her depression was exclusively the result of chronic pain and physical restrictions. The brave young man would have none of that. He replied, "No, Mom, I think you have been depressed for a long time, and the only thing that helped you feel better was exercise."

Kara still had work ahead of her, and so did I. She returned to normal life by accepting moderation and daily stretching, which had never been part of her aggressive fitness regime. Eventually, she was able to travel long distances to visit family, and she ran four miles per day five days per week. Four days per week she biked

20 miles and continued to incorporate the elliptical machine in her workout routine. That's still a whole lot of exercise—but it was a whole lot less for Kara.

As those improvements took hold and her lower spine loosened, it was time for me to address her rounded shoulders, forward-tilting head and the kyphosis that rounded her upper back. By increasing the strength of her abdominal muscles and trunk, her entire spine was liberated. As her posture improved, her mood improved dramatically, and she enthusiastically reintroduced her normal activities-with moderation.

Science Confirms the Body Mind Connection.

The link between posture and physical health is not an entirely new idea. As far back as the 1930s, Joel Goldwait, M.D., an orthopedic surgeon in Boston, shared many discoveries in his book *Body Mechanics in Health and Disease*. Yet much of his good work has been ignored or not actively pursued.

A skeptic might doubt that something so pervasive as depression, or even a problem limited to poor self-esteem, can be alleviated by improving posture. Yet Richard E. Petty, PhD., an author and professor of psychology at Ohio State University, is willing to accept simple, elegant solutions. In his opinion, it does not matter how the area of the brain that reflects confidence is triggered, as long as it is triggered in a positive manner. And his studies indicate that better posture gets the job done.

In association with Erik Pepper, PhD., an internationally known expert in holistic health and a professor at San Francisco State University, Petty wrote, in 2015, "Without teaching how to change body posture, only one half of the mind-body equation that underlies health and illness is impacted." Talk about a body mind miracle!

Pepper conducted an experiment that included one of his research students. She revealed that improving her posture also "improved my self-esteem, sense of empowerment, and reduced stress." She added, "…it proved the concept of health as a whole system between, body mind and spirit. When I listen carefully and act on it, my overall wellbeing is exceptionally improved."

Pepper, Petty and many others distinguished in their fields have conducted studies on this topic, and their research confirms what I have observed in my patients.

As mental health problems increase and damage more lives, young and old, and as economic pressures on getting great health care mount, we can no longer make the costly mistake of abandoning scientific evidence that provides cost-effective methods for conquering the invisible demon known as depression. *Standing up to depression* is one of them.

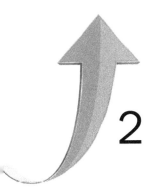

2

The Body Mind Miracle

As Dr. Keith Ablow so aptly stated in the foreword to this book, we have long understood the Mind Body connection: how our psychological state affects our bodily function. We are just now beginning to appreciate the Body Mind connection: how changing the body's physical state can positively influence our mental state. It is this Body Mind connection that adds valuable tools to target the intangibles of depression and relieve suffering.

I developed The Fairbend Method, a program of individual exercise, body mechanics and ergonomics, to teach depressed people how to train their bodies to overcome despondency, lack of motivation and low self-esteem. As I alluded to earlier in this book, my method helps people literally stand up to depression through the life skill of sound posture; it enables them to see, feel and understand how posture affects mood, and mood affects posture.

Physical therapy is widely understood as a way to address problems for patients with orthopedic problems and patients with other physical conditions, including cancer. However, the profession has neglected its powerful potential to address mental health issues and transform the prospects of patients with depression.

The most common physical symptoms depressed patients present with are neck, shoulder, arm and low back pain. Most often, these physical symptoms are related to poor posture. And posture is not only the basis of all motion, but also an unconscious expression of how we view ourselves. Thus, posture provides a unique doorway to the mind. The doorway works two ways (like all of them do). First, mental suffering can negatively influence posture. Second, poor posture can bring about more mental suffering.

The Fairbend Method program can help alter the negative mental loop that consistently and unconsciously tells a depressed person that the weight of the world is on his or her shoulders, that looking straight ahead is too frightening and that standing straight and strong against life's challenges is impossible. Improvements in posture set the stage for a depressed person to recover the mindset, confidence and attitude of the non-depressed person.

Through individual exercise, therefore, patients can improve posture and not only help prevent injury, but also increase energy, mood, self-esteem and productivity. To facilitate this transformation to the mindset of a non-depressed person, the patient must be aware of the restrictive mental habits they have adopted, but also the restrictive physical habits.

See it, Feel it, Understand it, Fix it

To reverse or eliminate the negative feedback loop of poor posture, the depressed person must first see, feel and understand what they are trying to change. The mind is the seat of consciousness and feeds the brain messages, both positive and negative, regarding emotions, posture and bodily position. The same mindset that affects posture influences processes like learning and reasoning.

Remember, many people who clearly demonstrate poor posture would never describe themselves as depressed, nor as even having poor posture. This is another reason the instruction "Stand up straight," usually spoken with frustration, doesn't work. Many people don't realize they are stooping or know what would enable them to change their depressed posture.

Emotion plays a part in an individual's ability to see a problem and be willing to change it. Eric Finzi, MD, PhD, calls this "emotional proprioception." The term proprioception describes both the conscious and subconscious sense of body movements and positions, which are determined by proprioceptors. Proprioceptors are message centers that are present in muscles, tendons, joints, the inner ear and other organs. These message centers receive and store information.

To help understand this concept of message centers, imagine having joint replacement surgery for a hip or knee. Since the artificial joint does not include living tissue, those areas no longer have the proprioceptors—which means that recovery must include redeveloping positive muscle memory in the muscles around the hip, knee, ankle and foot that contribute to balance and gait. The brain has to "recall" what it once knew for sure—how to move the lower extremity.

Learning sound posture through an individual exercise routine built on *seeing, feeling and understanding* takes into consideration the strong possibility that patients may not be fully aware of their physical presentation.

Seeing and Feeling...

Seeing and feeling the effects of poor posture may seem like an easy or obvious expectation. But the proprioceptors in a depressed person with poor posture have been collecting faulty messages and sending them to the brain. Poor posture comes to feel "correct" when it matches a person's internal emotional state. And habits are hard to change.

Depressed people who are not ready or able to make a change may say or imply, "This is who I am, leave me alone." This is often the message that depressed adolescents share, but is common in all age groups. The negativity is an expression of their depression, which they have yet to fully recognize and which may cause them to believe they are stuck with their condition.

This attitude may be hard for family members and colleagues to understand, unless they too have had personal experience with depression—whether as a parent, colleague, caregiver or medical provider.

"Wilma" is an excellent example. She had been suffering many physical problems and was depressed when she came to my office. As we stood together in front of a mirror, I began not with criticisms or by pointing out what was wrong. Instead, I said, "Wilma, ideally, we all would like our arms to fall at our side and our head to be above our shoulders. That's just natural. And together we can make that happen. Don't worry." Then we talked more about how we define sound posture, what it would look like and the effect it would have on physical comfort and function.

Wilma lit up and was eager to engage. At that point, I helped her stretch her shoulders and upper back for a few minutes before we took another look in the mirror. Sometimes a patient immediately sees a difference. Fortunately, that's how Wilma responded.

"Oh wow," she said. "I feel better that way, actually."

Her awakening, or disruption of negative muscle memories, felt like a door opening. Now we could proceed and expect to make some progress, because Wilma saw and then felt what we needed to correct. On her first visit, I recommended a few simple exercises she could repeat at home.

Understanding

At her next visit, I told Wilma that she appeared to be putting all her weight on her heels, which would normally cause someone to fall backwards.

"To counter-balance your body, you are throwing your head forward. The result is you can stand and walk, but not in a healthy way," I explained.

She understood immediately, visually recognizing the agonizing mechanics of her body. She came, she saw, but Wilma was not immediately able to correct the problem. Her muscles were tight, weak and sending incorrect messages about posture. By continuing to stretch those muscles over the following weeks, she gained the strength to make the adjustments and help the proprioceptors develop positive muscle messages and memories required for a healthy posture. Progress may seem slow at first, but imagine how Wilma enhanced her daily life by altering habits that had been causing her pain and limiting her enjoyment of daily activities.

Keep in mind that Wilma was a willing collaborator. Just doing the stretching exercises is not enough. For without the mind-body connection—seeing, feeling and understanding the process—posture and mood cannot significantly improve.

Secondary Improvements

In addition to improving posture, strength, flexibility and appearance, The Fairbend Method for Body and Mind also eliminates pain and secondary health problems. Success requires the patient to:

1. See and feel body posture as it is.

2. Understand the importance of achieving sound posture.

3. Feel improvement in mobility and strength of postural muscles with stretching exercises.

4. Recognize change in posture as a result of an appropriate and individualized exercise program.

5. Understand how these changes perpetuate themselves through body mechanics and sound ergonomics.

6. Feel a difference in an improved gait.

Since real change requires a concerted effort, almost all patients ask, "Is it ever going to become natural?"

Achieve the Life Skill of Sound Posture

My answer to the question above is always, "Yes, it will." As new habits develop, fresh positive messages are sent to the proprioceptors (those message centers in our bodies that tell us about how we are moving). Even if a person is not, at first, profoundly aware of postural improvements, they certainly notice the opposite—when they are lapsing into not standing upright. That feeling and acknowledgment alone is a big step. The individual then makes conscious adjustments, and the body begins to memorize a new way of being.

Although the steps to improvement described above seem simple enough, it can be difficult to fulfill these milestones with clients who have extreme physical and mental challenges. Let's explore a couple of case studies.

The Mind Teaches the Body

"Jason" became a patient when he was 14-years-old. He was over six feet tall, with a history of congenital heart disease and pulmonary stenosis. Jason had very poor posture attributed to his medical challenges and also suffered with extreme anxiety, which is common in patients with heart disease. Fatigue was also a factor.

Other challenges to treatments were his minor craniofacial symptoms, which minimized his facial expressions. He had difficulty describing what his body was feeling while exercising.

Jason's challenges became my challenge. How could I break through and better understand what he was feeling while exercising?

For months I asked Jason if he could *feel* a stretch we were doing and which I prescribed for him to do at home. "No, no," he would always answer. So, I changed my question and asked if he felt he was "working" while doing the stretch. He was able to answer that affirmatively. And, after a few weeks he volunteered, "Kathi, I can feel a stretch."

Jason finally had learned that the feeling of work was a stretch, and his new body awareness and proprioceptors connected with his mind. As the exercises strengthened his body and corrected his posture, he began to enjoy the way he looked and felt. According to his parents, Jason also began to correct his own sitting posture at home.

Another important addition to Jason's treatment had a profound positive impact on him—a specially trained service dog. This devoted friend enabled him to interact with and enjoy friends, school and some sports activities.

Able and Disabled

"Zena" is now 16, but she has been a patient since the age of 4. At birth she suffered a stroke and has left spastic hemiplegia, a neuromuscular condition in which the muscles on her left side are constantly contracting.

Like most of her peers, this very smart, high functioning young person is eager to learn how to drive and enjoy independence. Yet, she is also argumentative, with limited insight into how her negative attitudes and communication affects her physical success. Her poor mood and poor social and communication skills offend her peers. She blames her poor peer relationships on her disability.

Due to a difficult family situation, she spends most of her time with her devoted grandparents, who make sure she receives needed care.

Zena has dual perception as an able and disabled person. On one hand, she can strongly advocate for herself when at boarding school or camp. But she's inclined to use her disability as an excuse to avoid some activities.

In my office she presents as sullen, with her head down, and has a negative response to everything I suggest she could do to improve her abilities. For years, I have been asking her if she feels the difference when she walks well versus when she drags her leg, which she does not need to do. Mostly, she ignores anything and everything about her gait.

My approach now revolves around the Botox injections she receives to soothe the contractions in her arm and leg. My goal is to enhance the relief offered by this medication. At 16, she is finally able and willing to acknowledge that she feels a difference in her gait, but is skeptical about the positive mind-body connection the stretches and exercises are designed to improve, and, therefore, doesn't do them at home.

Many times, I have encouraged her to think and try to feel exercises and walking to engage her mind. I explain how thinking and feeling movement encourages muscles to work automatically, which would allow her to participate in activities with greater ease. Her response: "I don't get it." Her stubborn demeanor is relentless.

Sensory deprivation diminishes the proprioception in Zena's left arm and is a factor that limits her from initiating movement. She uses her left arm as a helping hand for her right side. She can tie her shoes one-handed! After a recent injection of Botox, the strength of her biceps enabled supination, a rotation of the forearm, allowing her palm to turn upward. I got excited when she could initiate the turning of her forearm and hand and urged her to use that motion.

Zena insisted that the muscles would never properly work. But by reiterating that the mind and body must work together, I taught her visual clues and patterns to practice the movement. Eventually, she began to show improvement, which created a positive feedback loop for more improvement. She now is able to put her arm on the steering wheel!

Where there is a will there is a way.

Human Touch

I'm not always the one encouraging better posture. For a year of Sundays, I watched "Theo," a gentle yet powerful businessman, shrink into himself, sitting in church with his head down, his body collapsed, his shoulders hunched. While sitting, he appeared to have difficulty breathing, and he was helped out of church before the service ended to avoid the crush of the congregation.

However, one Sunday Theo was at the end of the pew with three handsome grandsons sitting to his left. Behind him sat his wife and daughter-in-law, Alice. During the service, Alice reached forward and gently put her hand on Theo's shoulder. Soon he was sitting up with his back against the pew and his head above his shoulders. After communion he did not head out of the church but went back and sat in his pew, shocking his wife and Alice, who clearly were preparing to exit. After sitting and then kneeling, Alice continued moving her hand gently on her father-in-law's shoulder. By the end of the service, he was standing straighter and refused assistance when leaving church with the congregation.

It was a tender scene to witness. It revealed how kindness and human touch can profoundly affect posture and attitude. We all need help, in some form. Sometimes it is only a verbal reminder. At other times, it involves loving hands that assist physical and mental adjustments.

3

Spectrum of Depression

I mentioned that depression does not discriminate among, men, women, children, or by socioeconomic status. It can cause anything from mild disruption in life to complete devastation. The depressed population expresses itself in so many ways, including the basic categories, listed below.

Mild Depression:
Using the swimming pool as a metaphor, mild depression is in the shallow end. These are people who can function in society and participate in activities, but not always joyously. They can be friendly, even though they are not necessarily outgoing or sociable. Nor are they the kind of people who likely would call friends on the phone just to chat. The outreach is limited, because a shadow of darkness hangs over and subdues the mildly depressed. In fact, many people in this group and their family and friends may not relate their social reserve to depression. The mildly depressed may also be unable to relate their

physical symptoms of insomnia, fatigue or aches and pains to their depression.

This was the case with Conrad, whom we met in Chapter 1. He was concerned that his abdomen protruded and he insisted that weight loss was the answer. He had difficulty accepting that his protruding belly was related to his posture and mood. You might recall his multiple night time emergency room visits for chest and stomach pain, although each resulted in a diagnosis of anxiety (which so often accompanies depression).

Bipolar Disorder (formerly referred to as Manic Depression):

The deep end of the spectrum of depression includes severe conditions that are difficult to treat and may be lifelong issues. Bipolar disorder is one such severe condition. The traits of this unfortunate illness include extreme emotional highs (mania) and lows (depression), shifting from one to the other. The alternating extremes are often described as a roller coaster ride, though I would add that the ride happens while wearing blinders. The patient may not be warned when a fast turn or plunge will occur. Prescribed medications are often required to bring equilibrium to life. The patient with this illness at the extreme end of the spectrum must often cope with risky behaviors that can create mayhem with physical encounters and personal relationships. Suicidal tendencies and psychoses often accompany bipolar disease.

Major Depressive Episodes:

The category of Major Depressive Episodes rests in a wide middle range of the spectrum. I've mentioned it last because its characteristics are more common than you might expect and are often both visible and invisible to family, friends and colleagues of the afflicted person.

Note the use of "episodes" in this description. Fortunately, the people affected by this challenging condition are usually able to move through the depressive episode and finally recover.

Major depressive episodes also vary in degree and can affect people who are normally productive when they suddenly find they cannot function. They might watch Netflix all night, then be unable to get out of bed in the morning and go to work. Some may even be admitted to psychiatric hospitals for a short time.

Certain life struggles appear to elicit an initial episode or recurrence of depression more often than others:

- Complex grief after a death in the family is one example of the middle range. The complexity may be the result of guilt or feeling responsible for the death—emotional negligence, for example, or a feud that was never resolved.

- Loss of employment can cause a serious nose dive, because a job is part of a person's identity, not to mention financial well-being.

- A serious health problem can also be a trigger for depression, not only for the patient, but also for the caregiver of a seriously or chronically ill family member. Feeling helpless to improve the patient's condition can be cause for a depressive episode.

- Numerous medications warn that depression can be ignited as a side effect.

One more characteristic of the middle range is that depression can suddenly appear and can repeat itself years after recovery from the initial event. A song or anniversary may trigger memories of a lost love. A recurring health problem or a change in medication can send an otherwise stable person into a depressive episode as well.

Remember Kara, the fitness fanatic? Her episode was similar to others in this group who may self-medicate by taking up a strenuous fitness routine, which for a time may mask the depression. Who can fault the discipline of someone who runs five miles a day? They seem to be productive, but in truth they are running from their core problems, and the exertion they impose on their bodies may compound the problem.

Adolescents and young adults make up a niche group within the major depressive episode category. This group is sorely misinterpreted and often does not get treatment in a timely manner. Many parents don't recognize that their teenage son or daughter is suffering from depression. Instead, the uninformed diagnosis is, "Johnny's just being a teenager." Not necessarily. Take a look at the posture of Johnny or Janet. A child who suddenly is not him or herself, who slumps, curled up on the couch and stops communicating, is likely demonstrating angst and pain. Physical and mental wellbeing are intimately related and can often be associated with sedentary, sleep-deprived lifestyles, accompanied by social isolation produced by today's technology.

I urge parents to take these signals seriously. How many times have we read about a suicide or act of rage, and people close to the teenager say, "We had no idea!" Really? Pay attention. Poor posture, which may appear to signal nothing more than a failure to stand up straight, can actually be a profound message that things are not well.

Situational versus Recurring:

Depression can also be recurring or situational. Recurring depression might take the form of a seasonal disorder that afflicts people who cannot tolerate the darkness of winter. It may strike you as amusing, but some people may also be averse to a string of sunny days. They prefer variety in the weather, and, therefore, may avoid living in Florida or Southern California.

On the other hand, something like planning for a wedding of a son or daughter is rare and, therefore, situational. The preparation may have been a time of great enthusiasm, joyfully fulfilled when vows were exchanged. After the grand event there is an emotional let-down and emptiness, and this may lead to a depressive episode months later. Why? Because the focus and anticipation of the loving event are gone. A mom or dad might wonder, "Now what do I do with myself?"

Poor Posture Does Not Discriminate

There is a common denominator that ties together all these variations of depression: Mild or severe, <u>the posture of depression remains identical</u>.

Conrad the astronomer, who I place at the mild end of the spectrum, and Kara the fitness fanatic, who suffered a major depressive episode, each presented in the same way: Their shoulders slumped forward, with their heads in front of their shoulders. This is the fascinating aspect of poor posture: It does not discriminate.

The same was true for "Helen," despite the seriousness of her problems. When we first met, she presented in a humped state, with a forward-hanging head. Unlike other clients, she had an added layer of complexity called comorbidity, the medical term used to describe the presence of more than one disorder—physical, behavioral or mental. So, Helen's story can help us understand the challenge of balancing treatment for a patient with multiple diagnoses.

At the age of 54, Helen tripped over a rug and fractured her humerus, the large bone in the upper arm. She had surgery to insert a pin to hold the bone fragments together and promote healing. When that procedure failed, she underwent surgery for a total shoulder-joint replacement. That, too, was unsuccessful, and a year passed before doctors made a second attempt to replace the joint. This surgery was complicated by a complete tear of her biceps muscle and an overstretched brachial plexus (the nerve complex under the armpit). That adds up to three failed surgeries.

Helen was devastated because she did not have the use of her shoulder, arm or hand, due to weakness and pain. She experienced sensory deprivation and, therefore, lacked a sense of where her shoulder and arm were positioned. All these symptoms affected the function of her dominant right arm.

"I can't tell where my shoulder is, or where my arm is," she often complained.

I did my best to explain how nerves regenerate and assured her the brachial plexus problem would eventually heal. But she was so deeply depressed that she rejected the input and insisted, "I am disabled."

Helen had succumbed to her comorbidity. She could not separate her serious physical injury from depression, which put her toward the deepest end of the spectrum's middle range. Her condition made recovery extremely complicated.

By the time I met Helen, she was fearful of anything medical and afraid she might fall at any moment. She had been to several therapists in the previous two years and apparently had not experienced improvement since her last surgery.

Weakness in Helen's shoulder girdle contributed to her kyphosis (the forward curvature of her spine) and to the forward position of her head. She was deconditioned, with muscle weakness and tightness throughout her body. Over four years, it was nearly impossible to elicit any positive reaction, comment or physical sense that suggested she felt progress. Yet, in reality, there was huge improvement!

Finally, Helen noticed that her shoulders were open and not slumped forward, and her arms were hanging at her side, not in front of her body. Her changed appearance helped her develop an interest in life again and improved her attitude.

For example, after developing carpal tunnel symptoms and being in agony for six months, she agreed to a surgical procedure that dramatically improved the sensation, strength and dexterity of her hand. This allowed her to take part in more daily living activities, including cooking.

But one morning when I greeted her, instead of seeing improvements, her head was once again hanging, and her hands were clenched on her lap. She announced, "You are not going to be happy."

"Why? What happened?"

She had worried for years that she might fall again, and it finally had happened. She had tripped on a rug, again, and landed on the injured side of her body. The incident jolted her, and she knew something was wrong. Her arm wasn't hanging right.

"Well, if you had dislocated your shoulder you wouldn't be sitting there. There would be excruciating pain and a change in position of your shoulder. There may be some strain and bruising, but all your exercising and current improvement protected your arm."

I then pointed out that the reason her arm was in a different position was because she had returned to the bad habit of sitting with rounded shoulders and not using the muscles of her shoulder girdle to maintain her posture.

Although Helen had reason for concern—a fall could have created more problems—she completely recovered and began showing even more improvements. She resumed playing the piano at a near-concert level.

During one of our follow-up sessions, I couldn't resist telling her how great she looked. Her head was held high above her open shoulders and there was a smile on her face. Then I asked a tough question.

"Do you feel you have come out of the depression? I know the trauma of the initial accident and the changes that meant for your life were a massive stress."

She nodded. "I think the depression is gone."

I was thrilled and suggested that others would benefit from her story. By "others," I meant the millions of people who occupy a unique place on the spectrum of depression, and, yet, all share a common trait they may not be aware of—the possibility of recovery.

"You've come a long way, Helen."

To my surprise, days later I received a letter. It was hand-written with Helen's dominant hand, the one that had lacked sensation and functionality for so long:

> *So, when I am feeling down, my head is down and I feel small and hope no one is watching me. Now when I'm aware*

of this position, I look up and correct my position or just feel 'up' and then I feel better about myself. I also know that other people see this posture and see me differently than before. It is both a mood and self-awareness issue for me.

Physical Therapy for the Mind gives me a sense of my body in space, awareness of when some part of my body is 'out' and also what it feels like to be in a good place in my head and in my body. Having exercises to do gives me a feeling of control since there are so many parts of my injury that I cannot change.

Helen's recovery took a good deal of time, as the comorbidity was so restrictive. She was a prisoner of a vicious cycle: Her body was under terrible duress and, therefore, caused depression; or she was depressed and, therefore, could not be positive about the ability of her body to recover. Mind and body played at tag-team wrestling. When they both go negative, it's a tough duo to subdue. But it can be done. *That's what standing up to depression is a part of.*

The mental and physical connection evolved as Helen experienced small gains physically. She began to feel human, again, when she could take part in simple kitchen chores.

The harrowing self-fulfilling prophecy she had uttered— "I am disabled"—melted away and now she sits at the piano playing an entirely different tune.

Mood affects posture, and posture affects mood. It's a simple equation, but it is ignored far too often.

Depression is a disease like any other. It exists on a wide spectrum and can be treated, often with excellent results.

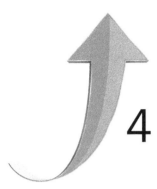

4

Secondary Health Problems

Posture is an unconscious expression of how we view ourselves. It is the basis of all movement, and, therefore, defines us when we walk, sit or stand. Depression remains invisible only when we refuse to look at and assess our bodies. So, let's define the most common secondary health problems, which are symptoms or additional diagnoses that accompany an initial diagnosis or can be caused by an initial diagnosis.

Poor mood causes poor posture, and poor posture causes poor mood. Each can be a secondary health problem to the other. However, poor mood creating poor posture can then also cause secondary orthopedic problems that include neck, shoulder, arm and back and foot pain, which can all negatively affect gait, balance, digestive and even breathing symptoms. Talk about a perfect storm of trouble. So, why would we ever ignore the way that posture is involved in it? That's the reason *standing up to depression* is so critically important.

Secondary Health Problems

Kara and Conrad, from Chapter 1, got their lives back by standing up to depression. Many more who suffer can be helped in the same way, but only if we begin to see the secondary health problems that often signal trouble.

Both these patients exhibited unsound posture in the neck, shoulders, back and arms. Millions of people are suffering from the same preventable issues. A slouching position often creates pain in the lower back area and can cause thoracic outlet syndrome, a group of disorders that may happen when blood vessels or nerves from a tunnel or opening below the collarbone and above the first rib (thoracic outlet) are compressed. Symptoms include varying degrees of pain, numbness and weakness in the entire upper extremity. This produces low mood, a decrease in energy, decreased productivity and low self-esteem. That makes sense, right? If the blood isn't flowing properly, there will be consequences.

How does thoracic outlet syndrome begin? Common causes include unsound posture, physical trauma from a car accident, repetitive injuries from job- or sports-related activities, certain anatomical defects (such as having an extra rib), scoliosis and kyphosis and pregnancy. Unfortunately, there are times when doctors can't determine the cause, but there is ample evidence that the body has been compromised.

Treatment for thoracic maladies usually involves exercise and pain-relief medications. Most people improve with these approaches. In some cases, however, you may not be able to avoid surgery.

Just as it did for Kara, the pain caused by prolonged poor posture can negatively influence thinking and decision making. As many studies reveal, therapy as described by The Fairbend Method can interrupt that downwardly mobile cycle by improving posture and setting the stage to recover the mindset of a non-depressed person.

Secondary Problems and the Spectrum

Secondary health problems can obscure the real problem. The patient arrives with complaints that he or she would never associate with the spectrum of depression, and yet …

One such indication of furtive depression is the manner in which a client reacts to discussing pain.

For example, I might ask,

"On a scale of zero to 10, how does it feel?"

Let's say the answer is 10 and that I then create an exercise plan based on that level of pain. If several visits later the answer is still 10, even though I see objective improvement and might expect a 7 or 8, this alerts me that dark moods are lurking beneath the physical symptoms. I then need to be asking questions to unearth a personal event or change that may have triggered depression.

What type of event or change of routine may be affecting their mood or self-esteem? Many men who come for treatment of an injury tell me about the athletic prowess of their youth. The loss of that self-image and ability can cause depression.

Another indication that the secondary problem is clouding the real issue can be when the client does not reduce prescribed pain medications, despite improvement. This does not always indicate a growing dependency on the drug. Instead, it may be due to an unwillingness to address the underlying emotions. For others, not reducing meds may be a matter of poor body awareness. Attention must be paid, or a problem will persist. Posture improves, and depression dissipates when we become more aware of our bodies. Posture affects mood, and mood affects posture.

Science Continues to Confirm that Posture affects Mood, and Mood affects Posture

Long-term effects of Unsound Posture

"Danielle" is a very smart 20-year old college student who I've known for a long time. She presented with a mild processing learning disability, accompanied by a four-year history of depression and an eating disorder that has required multiple hospitalizations. Her posture was unsound, with kyphosis from sitting in a twisted position for years. She arrived for her appointment and quickly declared, "I have a medical phenomenon."

I was eager to hear all about it, because I suspected this might be a clue to her underlying depression.

"Describe your pain," I said.

"Well, I have a pain that starts here—"

She touched the bottom of her sternum.

"—And it ends right here."

As she indicated her spine, I could barely suppress a smile. I'd known her long enough to feel comfortable risking a small joke.

"Whew, fortunately this is *not* a medical phenomenon."

"Really?"

She seemed a little disappointed, so I quickly explained.

"Your pain is the result of your poor posture, which for years has put pressure on your ribs. What you've described are the attachments of a particular rib."

"What do you mean, 'attachments?'"

"Well, as I've always said, our bodies are quite a contraption. Attachments connect one anatomical part to another. The front or anterior of the rib you are pointing at—is attached to the sternum, or breast bone by—"

"Duct tape?" she asked, with a smirk.

I smiled. "No, cartilage. And the back or posterior of the rib is connected to a thoracic vertebra, again with cartilage, fascia and tendon tissue."

"Sounds complicated."

"Yes, it is. When all the ribs are attached to vertebra, they make the ribcage which protects our lungs and heart. Then there is also muscle between each rib. So, Danielle, you can imagine if all these things are compressed because of poor posture, your energy and even breathing are affected. That's why you're in pain."

"Chain reaction."

"You got it."

As we talked, Danielle acknowledged that the pain was worse in the morning, yet she felt some relief during the day while she walked to class.

"Okay, that tells me that some soft tissue is involved and it's tender. Thankfully, your pain is mechanical in origin and can be resolved by—"

"Improving my posture."

"Right."

"I knew you were going to say that."

Secondary Health Problems

In fact, I'd been saying "that" for quite some time.

Danielle agreed that it was time to work on her posture, if only to ease her physical pain. I was delighted because our work would also improve the depression she presented. But, privately, I was astonished that not one of the many health providers she'd seen over four years for various ailments had suggested she improve her posture. For all this time her chronic physical pain had been preventable.

Am I criticizing all those highly trained and capable medical professionals? No, not really. Danielle's experience, however, does suggest that the link between posture and other ailments is still largely overlooked despite multiple scientific studies. Fortunately, breakthroughs are happening here and in other parts of the world.

The Psychiatry Profession Does Acknowledge a Posture-Mood Connection

The most encouraging report of how psychiatric professionals have begun to incorporate postural improvement when treating depressed patients was written in 2008 by Naomi Shraga, a London psychologist. She agreed to meet with a patient referred by a psychiatrist, because the woman had spent two weeks in Priory Hospital, with negligible results from medication prescribed for depression. "The patient and psychiatrist were willing to try anything," she wrote. By restoring a natural spinal position and balance, basically reeducating the body to maintain proper posture, the patient began to feel "... less vulnerable and better able to cope with her life's tension and anxiety." In short, the woman learned to stand up to her depression.

More proof came from a 2010 partnership between Columbia University and Harvard Business School. Researchers used saliva samples to prove that positive postures and "power postures" altered participants' hormone levels, decreasing cortisol and increasing testosterone. It is also well-documented that these two hormones influence disease resistance.

It should be noted that proper posture is dynamic, not static, and involves the movement of our bodies. "Power postures" are static because they are meant to be held for two minutes to make us feel more powerful, before entering a job interview, for example. The latter type is the result of research by Amy Joy Casselberry Cuddy, an American social psychologist. The term gained popularity after her TED talk in 2012, although it has also been called *"scientific overreach"* by some critics.

A more recent study published in March 2017 by Elizabeth Broadbent, PhD., Professor of Health Psychology, University of Auckland, and several colleagues, included observations of her own personality. One day while overcome by a "glum mood" she got relief after improving her posture. She concluded that if it worked for her it would work for others. And it did. The study, which included 61 participants, revealed that "upright posture [improved] affect and fatigue in people with depressive symptoms."

Achieving The Life Skill of Sound Posture

Let's get back to Danielle. If her attending physicians did not take note of her poor posture, a fair question is, what does sound posture look like? And how does someone like Danielle and the participants in various studies achieve it?

Remember, posture is the basis of all movement. Once the improved postures for standing, sitting and walking are learned, felt and visualized, human beings don't have to think about them. Sound posture is the proper relationship of body parts. Good habits become unconscious and repeat themselves. In short, it feels better when the body functions smoothly, and the mind embraces and memorizes the improvements.

Poor posture and poor health, on the other hand, are associated with the poor relationship of body parts and lousy body mechanics. Unfortunately, if we don't disrupt negative habits, they too become unconscious and limit our physical and mental competence.

A word of warning: Just as fitness fanatics can go to extremes with their exercise regimes, we would do ourselves a disservice if we begin to preach and reach the ideal posture. Joel Goldwait, M.D., the author and orthopedic surgeon I mentioned in Chapter 1, wrote that when discussing sound posture, it is important to recognize "that not all human beings are identical in their skeletal, muscular, neurological and pathological makeup."

This suggests that my ideal posture may be different than yours. This is obvious when we compare athletes, dancers or other performers. Certainly, there are similarities, and yet body types, personalities, postures and modes of expression vary. One common denominator can keep us focused: Mood affects posture, and posture affects mood. Have you ever seen an actor take a bow after a triumphant performance? Compare that to the baseball player who just lost the World Series and is walking to the losing team's locker room.

To objectify how you view your own posture, imagine the human body—your body—as a series of machines that are governed by the same laws of physics that affect machines of all kinds. Just as there is a cure for a sluggish automobile engine, dishwasher or elevator, there is a way to improve the mechanical performance of your body.

Part 2:
Learning The Fairbend Method to
Stand up to Depression

5

Ergonomic Health and Productivity in the Workplace are Influenced by Posture and Mood

We've covered a lot of ground in the last four chapters. We now know that posture is an unconscious expression of how we feel about ourselves, and we reveal those feelings whenever we stand, sit or walk. We also know that mood can be altered by improving basic mechanics of body movement. And we know that one picture-perfect posture does not exist because human beings are not born with the same physique or body type. There is also one more element that affects our ability to function: ergonomics.

Ergonomics is the science of how to use the body and to use equipment to perform a task without strain or injury. No doubt you are aware of increased concerns about carpel tunnel syndrome, hand and wrist injuries, spine injuries, blood clots and visual deterioration as a result of staring at computer screens for long hours. Fortunately, all these afflictions can be addressed when we accept that sound posture is the essential factor in battling ergonomic issues.

Ergonomics is not a new science, nor should sound ergonomics be thought of as a luxury in the workplace. Ergonomic health should be a priority everywhere, including home-office workspaces, nonprofit organizations and schools.

Technology in the workplace has created staggering statistics on musculoskeletal injuries. Fortunately, these data have been assessed by J. Paul Leigh, a professor of economics at San Jose State University and a research economist at Stanford Medical Center and the recipient of research grants from the National Institute for Occupational Safety and Health.

Leigh's published report estimates there are 8 million workplace injuries and illnesses costing billions of dollars annually in direct and indirect costs. The U.S. Bureau of Labor Statistics indicates that 17.3 percent of non-fatal work place injuries are due to musculoskeletal injuries of the neck, back and shoulders, and include tendonitis, thoracic outlet and carpal tunnel syndrome. Most of these injuries are due to poor working conditions and habits that lead to poor posture affecting mood and mood affecting posture.

Imagine a large group of workers in a single firm or business unaware their working conditions are taking a terrible toll on their bodies and minds. According to the journal *Burden of Musculoskeletal Diseases in the United States* (www.boneandjointburden.org/), half the American adult workplace population has suffered from one form or another of musculoskeletal disorder (MSD). The percentage for 65 and older workers jumped to nearly 75 percent. In 2012,

1 in 8 people of prime working age reported lost work days due to musculoskeletal conditions, for a total of 216 million days. I can't help but wonder how many of those injuries were secondary to depression. The negative statistics are increasing, as technology is affecting mood and posture and poor ergonomics.

Ergonomics

The word ergonomics comes from the Greek word Ergo, which means work, and it is the science of how a person uses a piece of equipment to perform a task without creating fatigue, stress or injury. Workplace musculoskeletal injuries are often referred to as cumulative trauma syndrome. Computer technology workers are not the first to experience these work-related problems, as they have been described as far back as the early eighteenth century.

Posture is the cornerstone of sound ergonomics, resulting in a decreased risk of injury while boosting productivity. I know you've now heard it many times from me: Posture affects mood, and mood affects posture. Ergonomic health includes both physical and mental issues. It's important to remember each individual plays a major role in any environment and is part of the solution for sound ergonomics.

Ergonomics is not a piece of equipment. *Nothing* is ergonomic in and of itself. Yet that doesn't stop many industries and professions from using the word ergonomics as a marketing tool (and it does sound good in a sales pitch for new office furniture). Buyer beware when drawn to an advertisement that says, "It's ergonomic!" Yes, there are faulty types of equipment, but they alone do not create faulty ergonomics in the workplace.

There are five critical categories in the science of ergonomics that are essential to the assessment of a worksite.

1. Biomechanical

Biomechanics is the science of how an individual uses the body to perform any task.

Evaluating the biomechanical aspects of a worksite requires accurate observation of how the body interacts with the actual worksite. Is the person being observed unable to sit in a neutral spinal position and work without stress or strain on the body?

A 6'3" man is not comfortable in a chair suitable for a 5 foot, individual. Nor is the 5' individual comfortable reaching for a desk that is 30" high and is suitable for a 6'3" individual.

Discomfort increases stress on the body, causing pain, poor posture and poor mood.

Posture is not static. It is dynamic and constantly changing. The efficiency of all movement is dependent on posture. This illustrates how critical posture assessment is regarding the mental health—mood—of the workspace.

The second factor in the biomechanical category is equipment, for it must be appropriate for the task and correctly sized for the stature of the individual.

2. Physiological

Certain medical problems or conditions can affect work posture and performance. These include hormonal imbalances, pregnancy, fatigue, age, poor nutrition, dehydration, arthritis and diabetes. Keep in mind each office worker is part of the solution for improving office ergonomics.

3. Psychological

Depression, secondary muscle stresses, strain and other illnesses can also occur from psychological factors, including lack of control over work demands and lack of job security, both of which can have a large impact on self-esteem. Boredom, as well as the daily burden of hostility from anti-social co-workers, are conditions that also need to be recognized.

4. Environmental

The physical conditions of the worksite, where one spends long hours, certainly matter. Is it too cold or too hot? Is the lighting adequate to illuminate work or is it too soft or too harsh, creating agitation while working? Is the worksite noisy from machinery, chatter among workers, or loud speakers? Clutter can also make an environment difficult to navigate.

5. Work Habits

There are more poor work habits than poor worksites. These work habits originate from poor posture and mood. Remember, poor posture affects mood, and mood affects posture. All poor work habits negatively impact the elements of ergonomics.

A few frequent poor work habits include: Sitting perched on edge of chair, legs crossed while sitting, reaching over papers at desk to key or just reaching up to desk to key, using poor lighting, holding the phone with one's head while typing (or "keying," as I call it), using monitors that are too low or too high or using multiple monitors placed too far apart.

Over time these poor work habits contribute to microtrauma due to increase in muscle tension and decrease in blood flow, causing a reaction from the entire musculoskeletal system. This problem is exacerbated by a combination of individual habits, such as inadequate breaks throughout the day or improper use of equipment, which may lead to poor posture.

Worksites: Business, Home and School

Many of the work-related problems physical therapists treat are caused by extenuated computer use. Computers are used in all industries, schools and businesses. It comes as no surprise that problems arise. Fortunately, there are safe ways to use your body both at home and at work to prevent and eliminate the postural problems related to using the computer.

Being fit to do a desk job may seem strange, but, in fact, a fit person can more easily endure daily work-related stress, such as anxiety from deadlines, long hours and unpleasant co-workers. However, many workers do little to improve the flexibility and strength needed for postural endurance of a work day.

Proper set up and use of the equipment provided is critical. How one uses the chair is as important as the quality of the chair. Lighting for an individual's worksite, the positioning of the keyboard and mouse, as well as the proper height of the monitor and the proper placement of paper documents, all affect posture whether sitting or standing, and therefore affect mood.

Proper computer posture enables you to sit with your spine in a neutral position, with your hips all the way back in the chair. Even chairs that are adjustable will not be much help if the worker's pelvis and hips are not situated over the central mechanism of the chair. This posture requires feet to be either flat on the floor or on a footstool that takes pressure off the spine. Shoulder blades should be touching the chair when using the keyboard. The head should be above the shoulders allowing the eyes to focus in the middle of the screen to eliminate any extraneous neck movement.

When using more than one monitor, each should converge in the middle of the work area and be slightly tilted in toward each other. The person, keyboard and monitors should be centered.

Frequent breaks are not only recommended, but essential, yet I find many workers refuse to take them for fear of underperforming, an example of a psychological factor where mood affects posture. In fact, there is solid scientific research that reveals sitting or standing in any one position all day is harmful to one's health. One solution is sit-to-stand equipment with electrically controlled legs that rise and lower a desktop to suit everyone's dimensions. This solution is very helpful whether sitting or standing, and far superior to the numerous sit-to-stand solutions that are placed on top of a non-adjustable desk.

The ideal position for computer screen is 90' to natural light. This isn't always possible, but is desirable.

Ambient light vs. fluorescent light directly over screen is preferred, and a task lamp to illuminate papers.

Changing the font and its size along with the brightness and color of background, is important to protect vision.

One size does not fit all. Depending on your height and body type, your worksite needs may be very different from that of a co-worker. The key is adjusting everything to enable healthy ergonomics.

When I do an ergonomic assessment for a corporation, small business or home office, observing employees' postures is a powerful way to determine the spirit and mental state of the overall environment. Postures that mimic depressed people shout at me. If too many individuals in a given office present poor posture, disturbances in workflow and sociability will certainly occur.

I often see that an individual is cramped, sitting on the edge of the chair, with shoulders rounded forward and often leaning to one side, with his or her head down. This position negatively affects breathing and results in a common complaint: "My neck and shoulders hurt, and the pain is radiating down my back." The individual also looks sad. Of course. How can a person smile when sitting in such an uncomfortable manner? It's a vicious cycle, demonstrated daily in our nation's largest corporations. These workers need to disrupt the cycle--by changing their position frequently, taking short breaks and, if they have a sit-to-stand possibility, using that option on a regular basis. Otherwise, they are doomed to hate their jobs and succumb to expensive and debilitating health problems.

Worksite Case Study

One bright and early morning I listened to a voice mail message from my contact at a law firm that specializes in insurance. I was asked to visit with an employee that needed an ergonomic assessment.

I knew Suzie, the employee, because I'd visited with her a few times before. This time she was complaining of back pain. As this satellite office was 100 miles away, my plan was to first call Suzie directly to discuss her problem. I asked her to send me photos of the way she works at her desk, because her verbal description would likely be inaccurate: employees can't watch themselves work.

"Suzie, it's Kathi Fairbend, the ergonomic consultant for your firm. I hear you're having problems again and requested a consultation."

"Yes. After I sit here at work for more than thirty minutes back fatigue forces me to stand."

I asked, "Are you working at a stand-up desk?"

"No. When I get up from my desk I just walk around and do different tasks until I feel better."

She confessed that the ordeal had decreased her productivity, and that her chair was 20 years old. That meant that this was only the second chair she'd been given during her 29 years working at his firm.

The pictures she sent confirmed what I already knew from previous visits. She was short and overweight, tilting toward the obese category. This made her unfit to be sitting 8 hours a day in a chair that was clearly too small for her stature.

"I want to be sure you get a proper chair, Suzie."

Suzie's back pain is an excellent example of how the physiological and biomechanical aspects of an assessment come into play. We could blame the old, inadequate chair up to a point. But a true reckoning cannot ignore the physical health of the employee. Suzie's weight was contributing to her pain and making it difficult for her to perform her job.

So, the next time you see one of those advertisements for "ergonomic" equipment, stop and ask yourself whether it is truly possible that a one-size-fits-all set-up will be right for each person in the office. Not likely.

The five essential elements of an ergonomics assessment give you the best chance to tailor a healthy home office or employee workspace. Many companies benefit from a brief seminar that helps the entire workforce, management and employees, to grasp the importance of sound ergonomics. The more individuals and levels of management that understand these principles, the more successful their company will become in achieving ergonomic health. Productivity and morale will naturally improve when the mood in the environment is established by people with healthy postures.

6

Developing Individualized Exercise Programs

The goal of each individual exercise program is to teach the life skill of sound posture that improves mood and health and the ability to stand up to depression. The depressed patient's call to request an appointment or phone consult with me as a physical therapist is usually due to musculoskeletal pain and not depression. It is unusual for depressed patients to say they are depressed and they most likely have been hesitant to make the call. I try to gain some insight as to "why" they are seeking an appointment and instill some thoughts about their posture, related to their problem, by asking if they have any neck or back pain related to the reason for their appointment. As the patient is the major part of solution, I feel this helps them feel invested before the first appointment. Depressed patients often resent their pain and need "hands on" care and reassurance that they have made the right call. It's part of my challenge, when starting to help a depressed patient, to detect their inability to either recognize or feel comfortable acknowledging their depression.

Individual Program to Stand up to Depression with the Body Mind Connection

The initial appointment provides patients a chance to tell me about themselves, their activities, health histories and what prompted their call. It's my responsibility to listen intently to the patient's life challenges in order to guide them to meet their needs and responsibilities and to enjoy life.

This initial visit also provides an opportunity for me to observe body awareness, posture and movement patterns, which most likely are impaired. If patients are depressed, these body postures most often look like the unconscious and harmful posture previous described in Chapter 4: Secondary Health Problems. These secondary health problems usually signal trouble. I often ask patients if they think their posture has changed since they developed the problem they are experiencing.

Frequently, individuals will say "I know I have bad posture," to which I respond, "Do you think that is true or did someone tell you that?" *The response is often an indication of their own body image, rather than reality.*

Frequent clues that depression is the problem are how long they have had the same problem and what they are currently doing (or not doing) to correct the problem. As an example, a person may come in with persistent neck, shoulder and/or arm pain with no known cause and no attempt at treatment. It is not uncommon for some individuals to have delayed making an appointment even though an orthopedic physician may have recommended physical therapy 4 to 6 months prior. Others have been to multiple therapists and were never able to follow through with the program, which had been too expensive and time-consuming or required multiple appointments. Others were never given any or were given insufficient instructions to follow at home. All of which I completely understand!

I explain The Fairbend Method of individual exercise is designed to teach the life skill and exercise regime without multiple visits, where consistency is the key factor, not length of time spent daily. The program is designed to enable consistency by *incorporating* it into a person's daily life, making it possible to do the exercises anywhere without special equipment or location. The program should serve as a warm up and cool down for cardiovascular activates.

Depressed patients will undoubtedly say a specific neck, back or shoulder problem is the reason for the appointment and display obvious resentment about the pain and the need to seek help. I do reassure them that the first objective is to overcome the pain. If patients are not forthcoming about their depression, they are not usually forthcoming about the reasons for the originating pain. Despite this, the presentation of the symptoms and history indicates that depression exists. This is where the invisible and visible signs begin to collect and gives clues to their health.

Secondary Health Problems Signal Trouble

Teenagers need reassurance to feel at ease, and I often ask if they "feel they have been sent by someone else," which usually brings a smile, as with Lucy, a tall overweight girl who dragged herself into the office. Her expression prompted me to smile and ask "Do you feel like you have been sent here, rather than your deciding to come here?" She picked up quickly, smiled and said, "Yes."

We then spoke about her activities which included many hours sitting in the middle of the bed to do homework, occasionally going to the gym to use the elliptical machine. She informed me that she had no intention of doing any exercises. I asked if she thought she was depressed. "I guess so. Too much school work, too many college applications, no social life—and I babysit all the time." She concluded with, "That's the deal." I explained mood affects posture, and posture affects mood, and that it could be the cause of the painful dowager's hump that prompted her mother to make an appointment for Lucy to meet with me.

Lucy was interested in the posture and mood relationship. But her mother was not! I taught her two simple stretches that she agreed were doable. A BEGINNING. This was a double visible invisible situation…. for neither the mother or daughter could see the originating cause of her pain.

Changing Posture is a Process

After clarifying a patient's physical history and any past possible injuries, the opportunity is open for the patient to start their individualized exercise program. The hands-on approach of The Fairbend Method is to relieve pain by developing and integrating sound postural patterns which will help improve and eliminate pain and improve mood.

This is my opportunity to explain that posture is basic to all exercise programs and basic to all movements from walking to performing at the Olympics. I never tell anyone to change their posture, until they see, feel and understand the undesirable posture that is creating their pain. This involves exercise to enable the mind to provide messages to their brain and body. When flexibility, strength and visual clues work together, patients see and feel what posture they can achieve to relieve pain and prevent new pain and or injury. At this juncture patients (like Wilma in Chapter 2) are able to

Developing Individualized Exercise Programs

understand the posture and mood, and mood and posture, connection. Exciting for both of us!

The Fairbend Method underscores that exercise instruction requires a pleasant and appropriate setting—the experience should be enjoyable and a process that **starts at the beginning and not with the end product.** An analogy I often use is that you can't fix the chimney if the foundation of the house is crumbling, so, we, too, need to start with the basics.

An exercise program is only as effective as the position the person is able to assume to perform the exercise correctly. The visible posture of the depressed patient indicates their inability to control their posture against gravity. Lying down is a starting position where most people have some sense of control over their body parts. Teaching muscle relaxation techniques first is often necessary to prevent accessory muscles from interfering with specific muscles or movements.

When the person lies down, I encourage them to allow their body to settle, to picture and elongate their spine from one end of the room to the other. All exercises should be done in a slow and deliberate manner, with the understanding that feeling a stretch is OK, but feeling pain is never OK.

You will find the exercises and instructions in the next chapter (Chapter 7). I suggest that patients start their home program and spend at least five minutes a day with just the first four or five exercises to provide consistency and eliminate pain. The daily routine ensures the next session will be more valuable. Depending on what method the patient thinks will work best for their home program, it can be written with or without diagrams and personal pictures or videos on a smart phone and iPad. For some accountability I might ask the 9 to 14-year-old children to text "done" after their daily routine. I have one distracted psychiatrist that uses texting "done" to me, just for her own accountability.

Each individualized visit is designed to build on the basics, ending with a program that is 10 to 15 minutes long as a life-long daily regime. I spend time working with the depressed patient to figure out where and when they will do the exercises, usually in combination with some other activity that is already part of their routine. Of course, we can make the program longer; realistically, however, individuals will no spend more than 15-20 minutes on a daily basis. Consistent daily stretching keeps the mood and posture, and posture and mood, model firmly entrenched in the mind, providing messages to the brain. Patients become enthused to see that when the appropriate exercises are precisely done, it take little time and effort to produce results.

Exercise - A Life Routine

The goal for all human beings is mobility, strength and, then endurance. Without this triad, we cannot balance or do aerobic exercises or train for the Olympics. Exercise is the only way to achieve these goals.

Pain is often a great motivator. My patients realize that they will never have relief unless they learn to exercise and strengthen the posture-mood connection, which in turn will improve body mechanics, ergonomics and mindset. Also, the exercises must become habitual and performed at home, not just in my office. Chapter 7 introduces the types of exercises and stretches I recommend in the early and advanced stages to achieve sound posture-The Body Mind Miracle. Everyone's program includes gait training, as gait is affected by faulty postures. Each individual has unique challenges, requiring a customized plan. The reader will see that the exercises are set up and described from basic and easiest, then progressing to more difficult, with explanations that will advise what one should and should not to feel and how to see improvement. There's also advice about some "not to dos," for particular problems.

Essentials of The Fairbend Method

The MIND is responsible for learning and connecting emotions with sound posture and helps reinforce and perpetuate that posture. Posture, dynamic not static, reinforces how we use our body, and The Fairbend Method addresses this through detailed instructions and practice in Body Mechanics. This efficient movement allows essential muscle groups to work while others relax. In addition to Body Mechanics, which allows for an efficient and pain-free gait, The Fairbend Method provides instruction in sound Ergonomics, wherein one incorporates body mechanics to use their body and equipment (for example the desk or lap computer or smart phone) to perform a task without stress strain or injury- *posture being the essential factor in sound ergonomics*. Sound ergonomics helps individuals avoid injuries such as carpal tunnel syndrome, spinal injuries, thoracic outlet syndrome, vision problems and even blood clots. The depressed are more prone to such problems due to their lack of movement in prolonged awkward positions and their mood and posture and posture and mood when performing activities.

The following chapter will provide specific exercises that will help everyone Stand Up to Depression. Enjoy!

7

Exercise Instructions to Improve Posture and Mood and *Stand Up to Depression*

The previous chapters have discussed the body connection to sound posture---the idea that posture affects mood and mood affects posture. Sound posture is a life skill easily learned with an individual exercise program. This approach enables each individual with unique challenges due to overall health, previous injuries and depression to work on the triad of mobility, strength and endurance necessary for pain relief, sound body mechanics, sound posture and enhanced mood. In other words, it is necessary in order to *stand up to depression*.

Let's Get Started

With any new exercise regime, be sure to check with your physician before beginning.

Exercise Instructions

The program starts with basic exercises to mobilize and feel the neutral position of the spine. Once these are understood, felt and performed effectively the routine can be expanded by increasing the difficulty and to accommodate particular interests and participation in activities. The key is consistency. Try to find a time of day or another activity that seems a natural fit for a period of exercise.

If helpful take notes.

Begin with Very Basic Exercises

The exercises should be relaxing and enjoyable. Try to keep your eyes open to both see and feel what you are doing as you think of where the action occurs. Technique is more important than result. Results will follow technique.

Starting Position:

- Lie on ground or floor with both knees bent and feet flat on floor. (Bed is OK if one has extreme muscle tightness or feels too vulnerable to lie on floor due to depression.)

- Arms straight at side with palms up.

- Allow your back to "<u>settle</u>" when you first lie down.

Picture you your shoulders and hips like the wheels on your car-firmly on the ground.

1. Low Back or Lumbar Stretch

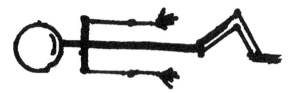

- This exercise is the starting position for all exercises.

- MOST IMPORTANT this exercise allows your spine to be in neutral. The position for all activities including standing walking and sleeping.

- Gently pull in low deep abdomen-do not use hips and do not push back down.

- Imagine your back 10' long with shoulders as far apart as possible. Allow shoulder blades to slide together under your back.

- Without lifting head aim your forehead for your knees.

- Try to feel a stretch somewhere-- hold slow 5 counts- relax repeat 5 times.

If you don't feel a stretch somewhere, pull low stomach in lower, deeper, longer.

Allow your shoulders to go further apart as you aim forehead for knees.

You may not see your knees until you have done the exercise for several days. Ideally, your head will rest on the base of your skull.

If your neck is particularly tight-- do not hesitate to use a small towel under your head and neck--not your shoulders.

Exercise Instructions

2. Arms as Arrows

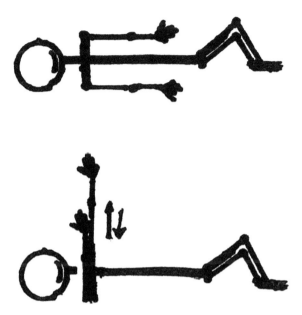

Shoulder motion and neck motion are closely connected to the ability for one's head to be ABOVE the shoulders, for sound posture. A key to the Body Mind Miracle is this position of your neck and shoulders.

This exercise should help you feel the back of your shoulders firmly on the ground and your shoulder blades firmly underneath your back.

- Starting position is the same as exercise #1. Take time to make sure your low, deep abdomen is engaged, your back feels long, your shoulders are broad, with your forehead aimed toward knees.

- With the back of your shoulders firmly on the ground, keep your elbows straight and reach with straight arms straight up to ceiling. Pause--

- Picture your arms as arrows, reaching up, staying straight, as you use your shoulders to pull your straight arms (do not bend elbows) down into the ground, as you squeeze shoulder blades together.

- Try this with your palms facing you.

- Then with palms turned away from your face.

- Then palms facing your face.

    Repeat 3 or 4 times in each direction.

Exercise Instructions

3. Knees Toward Shoulders

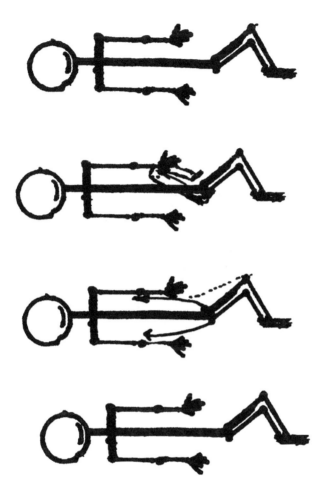

This exercise will help stretch the long muscles from the base of your spine to the base of your skull. It will also help to stretch some of the gluteal or buttock muscles.

- Starting position is the same as exercise # 1.

- Gently use hip to raise one knee at a time up TOWARD your chest.

- Aim the knee toward the shoulder on the same side. Then bring the second knee up from the hip toward chest, also aim that knee for the same-side shoulder as the knee you have brought just brought toward your chest.

- Be particular to keep the hips and pelvis on the floor and allow hips to roll up. Hold 5 counts.

- Expect to feel a stretch somewhere in your spine and maybe between your shoulder blades and neck.

- It is safe to put hands under thighs—not on knees or lower legs—to support legs while you enjoy the stretch.

- Then using your hips, lower one leg at a time, returning to the starting position, with feet flat on floor and close to hips.

- Repeat 2 or 3 repetitions.

4. Shoulder and Upper Back Stretches

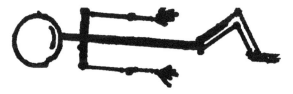

Keep in mind SOUND POSTURE enables your head to be above your shoulders. The key to defeating depression is most often in your neck and shoulders.

4A. Fingers on Shoulders

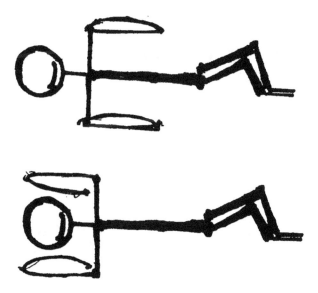

- Starting position as in exercise #1.

- Keep shoulders firmly on the ground.

- Bend elbows to *allow* fingertips to gently touch the top of your shoulders.

- Roll shoulders into the ground-until your fingers touch the ground behind you-pause--- your elbow will rise toward ceiling as shoulder rolls back.

- Then roll shoulders back down to ground, until upper arm is again against the ground.

- Be slow and deliberate as the shoulders do the movement.

- 4 or 5 repetitions is adequate

4B. Fingers on Shoulders

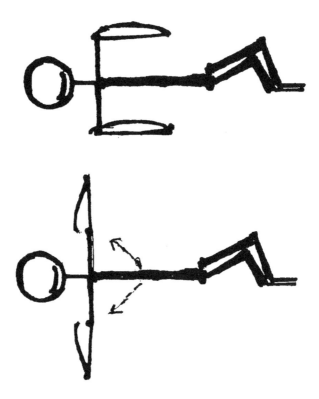

- Next, with your fingertips still gently on top of your shoulders as in 4A.

Exercise Instructions

- Stay on the back of your arms with fingers loosely on top of shoulders.

- Upper arm should be close to upper body.

- Slide your shoulders on the back of your arms-- out to side--to level of shoulders. Keep the back of your arm on the ground.

- Use inside of shoulders to pull shoulders and upper arm back to side.

- Keep in mind shoulders do the work.

- 4 or 5 repetitions is adequate.

5. Drop Both Arms Straight Back Over Head

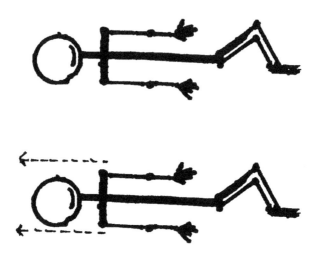

- Starting position same as Exercise #1

- Raise arms from shoulders, keeping elbows straight, allow straight arms to go back over head. Do not worry how far back your arms go, pay more attention to keeping your elbows straight to insure shoulders do the work.

- Be particular to notice, the farther your arms go back the easier it is to aim forehead toward your knees and to see them.

- You will feel a stretch in the back of your neck as your arms go back-and

- You will feel the muscles in the back of your neck working/strengthening as you slowly bring your arms back down to your sides.

 Be sure to use your neck and not your jaw.

- 4 or 5 repetitions is adequate.

6. Alternate Straight Arms Over Head

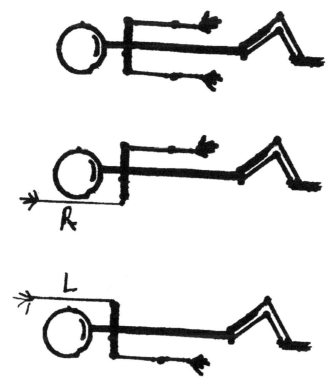

- Starting position as in Exercise #1

- Using shoulders and keeping arms straight alternate each arm up and over head.

- It is more important to keep the elbows straight and use the shoulders to do the motion than to have wrists resting on the ground when your arm is overhead. As you gain mobility in shoulders and upper back, your wrists will touch the ground.

- 4 or 5 repetitions each side is adequate.

7. Alternate Sliding Each Leg Out Straight

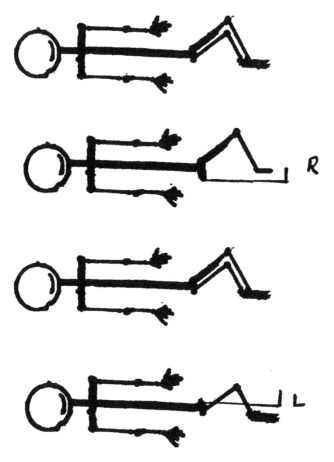

- Starting position as in Exercise #1

- Keep heel on the ground and use your hip-buttock, gluteal muscles to alternately push/ slide each leg out straight, then pause.

- Keeping heel on ground, use posterior hip muscles to bring leg back up to starting position with foot flat on the ground.

- 4 or 5 repetitions each side is adequate.

Exercise Instructions

8. Opposite Arm and Leg

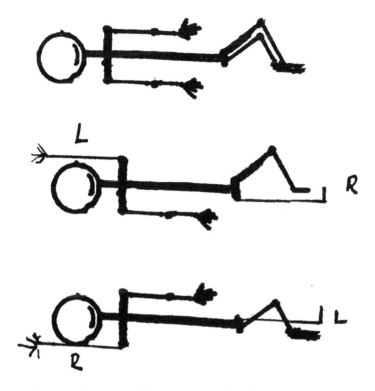

Spend time with this exercise, for there are many large muscles of your legs, back and arms working to both stretch and strengthen.

This exercise is a very functional way to strengthen abdominal muscles as they engage though out the exercise.

In addition, if you have a scoliosis this exercise will help stretch the convex or outward portion of your spinal curve.

- Starting position as in exercise #1.
- Alternate straight arm overhead and opposite leg out straight.

- Right arm will be over head and left leg will be out straight.

- Left arm will then be over head, and right leg will be out straight.

- Use the same technique to raise arm and slide leg as in exercises 6 and 7.

- This is a normal motor pattern and the pattern of normal gait.

- Work up slowly to 10 repetitions on each side.

Exercise Instructions

9. Butterfly and Picture Frame

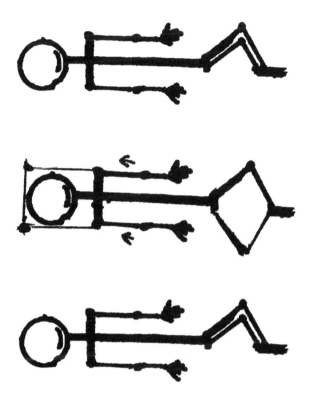

- Starting position as in exercise #1.

- With feet flat together on the ground, slowly *droop* your hips out to the side. Do not use your knees. Let gravity help feel the stretch of the inner thighs and hips.

- Be particular to have the soles of your feet together when

  Your hips are drooped out to the side.

- At the same time, hold your elbows, not forearms, and use shoulders to allow your arms to drop overhead. They may not go to ground until you have had some practice.

- Hold the position for 20 seconds, then relax to starting position and reverse your hold on the elbows and droop hips out and arms overhead again. One time your right arm will be closer to the ground and the next time the left arm will be closer to the ground.

- Holding your elbows makes a square— the picture frame. Your head is in the middle. You are the picture.

- Do 2 or 3 repetitions.

10. "E- W" Exercise

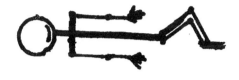

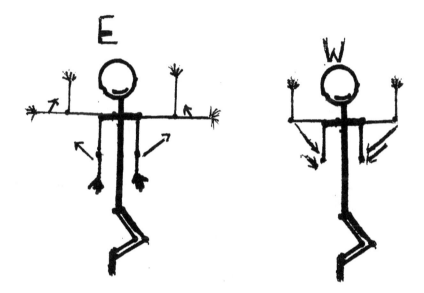

This exercise will improve upper back mobility and shoulder rotation. As mentioned, this movement is critical to enable your head to be over shoulders and to stand up to depression.

- Starting position as in Exercise #1. By now I'm sure you feel that pulling in your abdomen, broadening shoulders and aiming forehead toward knees is natural.

- If you feel that your head will rest comfortably on the floor, you could remove the towel, if you have been using one, and feel if you are comfortable without the extra support.

- Lie on back and place your arms out to the side, at shoulder level.

- Then bend elbows and allow your hands and fingers to drop back to floor ((Diagram 10 E)

- For some individuals this position alone will produce a stretch in chest and shoulders.

- Your arms will be a right angle to your body with your head the middle portion of an uppercase E.

- Keep your fingertips, shoulders and shoulder blades on the ground and slowly squeeze your shoulder blades and pull shoulders and elbows toward your side, forming a W.

- Pause and then squeeze shoulder blades and slide back to E position.

- When your arms will come in close to body—

Try the E to W exercise standing as a way to build more strength in upper back.

When standing be particular to keep head over shoulders.

3 or 4 repetitions is adequate.

11. Hamstring Stretch

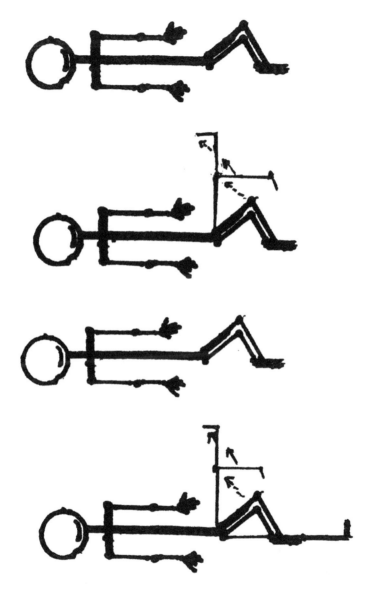

There's an adage that people with tight hamstrings always have neck and low back pain, and people with neck and low backpain always have tight hamstrings.

Why?

Tight hamstrings prevent sound posture and stress our spine---- and these are the first muscles to involuntarily tighten, for protection, when one has low back or neck pain.

- Starting position as in Exercise #1.

- Bring one bent knee up over hip.

- Then try to straighten knee UPWARD toward the ceiling.

- When you feel a stretch in the back of your thigh, and your leg is as straight as possible, (with knee over hip).

- Then bend ankle straight toward you and pause to help stretch calf.

- It is important to stretch. Do not straighten without feeling stretching in the back of your thigh.

- There is no need to hold leg with hands. Keep hip and pelvis on the ground.

- One should not feel discomfort in back or neck- stretch but no discomfort.

- Alternate legs.

- 4 repetitions but hold at least 10 seconds.

- If each leg will assume a right angle --- then progress to sliding the opposite leg out straight while holding one leg up straight.

- Keeping your eyes focused on the knee that you are straightening will encourage your posterior neck muscles to strengthen.

12. Hip Flexor Stretch

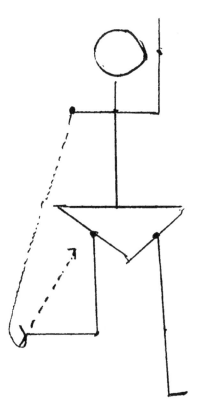

This exercise requires standing. It incorporates the mobility, strength, control and balance of your spine and the posture acquired from the previous exercises.

The hip flexor group is the opposing group to the hamstrings and often creates a torque or twist and pain to our spine when tight. Unsound posture and sitting for a prolonged period often result in tight hip flexors and the inability to Stand Up to Depression.

- I suggest facing and standing close to a wall to start.

- With one hand on the wall and straight up to ceiling, keep the leg on the same side as your arm is up the wall, still and straight.

- Then move the other leg straight back from the hip.

- And next bend the knee on that leg up, and try to hold your foot, preferably at the toes. If you cannot hold the foot, then pause and slowly lower leg. Alternate legs.

- If you can hold your foot, the object is not to pull your foot to your hip, but instead to allow your knee to *droop* to the ground, as though you were holding the leg in a sling.

- You would like to feel the stretch in the front of your thigh.

- Alternate legs

- If you are nowhere near reaching your foot- you can back up to a chair or stairs and put your foot on the chair or the second step while you stand straight and hold the railing or chair in front of you.

- Practice will help!

    Starting the routine is simple and you might find additional guidance from downloading my DVD Stretch Away Back Pain from my website www.ergoworkplace.com.

    I am also available by phone for consultation.

8

Maintaining Sound Posture to *Stand Up to Depression*

It is always a joy for me to help one more person stand up to depression! Each patient is equally upbeat, because he or she is healthier in mind, body and spirit, and each enjoys the priceless bonus of improved appearance. The correction in posture not only helps each person maintain positive mood, self-esteem, self-confidence, increased energy and productivity, it also means the individual is more likely to make sound decisions—based on confidence and optimism—in all aspects of life.

Standing up to depression is a life skill. It must be practiced and maintained. As with any illness, people who have overcome depression will benefit from an occasional checkup. As individual exercise is a vital modality necessary for the treatment of depression, I encourage my patients to come back for a "tune-up."

Continued practice of the exercises is important as it helps each person to become more proficient and reap further benefits each time an exercise is performed correctly. This makes it possible to expand the basics of their initial individualized plan without adding time to the daily regimen. As one becomes more mobile and makes it a habit to employ sound body mechanics and ergonomics in the office and at home, each person gains strength. Then, at the time of the follow-up visit, we can discuss how to improve techniques, as well as add, subtract or intensify exercises.

Also, when depression is minimized, many people show more interest in different types of activities. To be able to fulfill those wishes without risk of injury, more mobility and strength may be needed. Again, this is what makes the program described in this book unique. It is a method designed to *expand* quality of life. The practice of standing up to depression is similar to learning and mastering a sport, such as golf or a musical instrument. In fact, the daily exercise routine provides a good warm up and cool down for cardiovascular activities.

Life happens. As seasons change, we alter our schedules and activities. The back-to-school ritual may take a toll, as does the end of the school year when parents scramble to make summer plans. Starting a new job, moving, holidays, planning a wedding, becoming pregnant and giving birth—all these events affect mind and body and can derail an exercise routine. Yet, the busier we are, the more we need a healthy program. Otherwise, regression may set in and not be noticed by the individual. This is another reason for follow-up visits. I'll notice changes, be able to re-establish correct posture before regression in their illness and reestablish additional visits to prevent a downward slide. I'm usually quite busy during holiday seasons, because "life happens." In fact, the people who struggle the most with depression will come once a month for years

Maintaining Sound Posture to Stand Up to Depression

to check themselves. The visits allow us to talk about the struggles they have had, and also anticipate and prepare for the impact of coming events. The goal is to keep standing up to depression!

Fortunately, technology has enhanced how we all communicate. Email, texting, faxes, smart phone images and personal videos can all be harnessed so that the information contributes to the maintenance of good posture and mood. Even so, I encourage patients to keep appointments even when they believe they are doing fine. Calling me with a quick question, hoping to resolve a minor complaint over the phone is possible, if I have a recent (in person) postural reference.

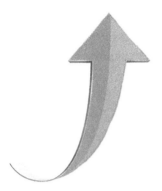

Afterword
Believing in Simplicity

    Believing in simplicity is difficult for some people. Fortunately, there is ample scientific research to support The Fairbend Method, which proves that adjusting posture can have immediate positive results and, in some cases, actually reverse depression.

    In a fast world, full of new pharmaceutical discoveries, gadgets, theories and technologies, the reader is reminded that much of what Stand Up to Depression teaches is based on information that was discovered in the early 20th Century. Society simply did not grasp its significance then.

    Now we have the chance to improve our lives —if we'll just believe what we see in the mirror.

—Kathi

About the Author

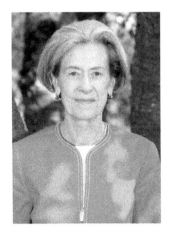

Kathi Fairbend, MS, RPT, developed The *Fairbend Method of Physical Therapy for The Mind* through her extensive clinical observations and teaching experiences. Her crucial insights into the connection between depression and improved posture have since been verified in various scientific studies.

The physical therapist's expertise in ergonomic health and the prevention of cumulative trauma syndrome resulting in computer-related injuries, which include back and neck pain, have been presented in health articles and business journals. Her work is also the subject of a PBS *This Old House* episode, which features the home exercise space she designed with an emphasis on the importance of effective stretching in cardiovascular exercise.

Fairbend is also a groundbreaker. As the producer of *Total Hip Replacement*, a film about pre-and post-treatment for total hip replacement surgery, she was the first American physical therapist to introduce her treatment program about this critical topic before the National Physical Therapy Conference.

A proponent of visual media education, Fairbend is the producer and featured instructor in *Stretch Away Back Pain* and *Stretch Away Neck, Shoulder, and Arm Pain* videos included in a growing series of DVD presentations.

For ten years, the graduate of Boston University (MS) and Tufts University (BS) has been the ergonomic consultant for the Wyss Institute for Biologically Inspired Engineering at Harvard University. She advised architects and interior designers and has consulted with administrators and faculty to create a sound ergonomic work environment. In a decade, the number of people she cares for at the institute has expanded from 50 to more than 400. The mission ranges from providing weekly ergonomic adjustments for individuals for injury prevention to helping individuals resolve musculoskeletal and physical problems related to work and elsewhere.

The breadth of her consultation services is a long list of vital institutions, such as the Department of Health, Education, and Welfare, and Dedham Medical Associates, where she helped establish and design its first physical therapy department. Other clients include the New England Heart Center, Donovan Leisure Newton and Irvine, and various educational facilities, such as Dartmouth Medical School, not-for-profit groups like the Foundation for Informed Medical Decision Making, and a wide range of corporations.

As an expert witness in courtroom litigation, she has seen the dramatic and debilitating impact of poor ergonomics. Her writings

About the Author

draw from these experiences to express the human cost of poor posture and depression often influenced by work environments.

Fairbend has been named a Life Member of the American Physical Therapy Association, has ties to the American College of Sports Medicine, and has taught at Northeastern University's Bove College of Health Sciences, Boston University, Simmons College, and Babson College, where she also became an advisor for the entrepreneurial program.

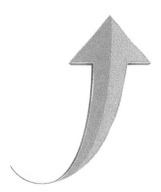

Acknowledgements

Stand Up to Depression could not have been written without patients who trusted me not only to help them with their physical problems, but also shared their struggles with depression and were open to the notion that the work we were doing could benefit their bodies and their minds. I am profoundly grateful to have had the opportunity to help each and every one of them who regained their physical and emotional strength--- who "stood up to depression."

My colleague, mentor and friend Keith Ablow, MD deserves praise for his steadfast enthusiasm and encouragement for me to pursue writing Stand Up to Depression. Keith contributed the foreword and clearly understands the role physical therapists can play in identifying and helping depressed patients. He urged me to get the word out to as many of those patients, and as may physical therapists, as possible.

It was a delight to work with my editor Sharyn Kolberg. Her warm enthusiasm about Stand Up To Depression, along with her pertinent edits, helped clarify my message.

Acknowledgements

Finally, I wish to acknowledge Karen Lacey and Douglas Glen Clark, who provided expertise and consultation about the book's premise and relevance in today's culture. They helped galvanize my intention to keep writing and to bring this project to fruition.

PTM©
PHYSICAL THERAPY FOR THE MIND

Since 1963, my private practice of physical therapy and ergonomic consulting has taken me from treating patients in the projects of Mission Hill, Boston, MA to board room presentations, expert witness testimony in courts and work at the White House, Washington, DC. I have witnessed all the evolving trends in medicine and health care, as well as evolutions in diagnoses, types of injuries and illnesses, methods of treatment and use of technology.

Throughout, my passion has remained prevention and patient education, through individualized one-on-one treatment.

I founded the specialty PTM—physical therapy for the mind—to address the dramatic rise in the numbers of depressed individuals. Physical therapists are ideally situated to recognize depression and institute what I call *body-mind treatment plans* designed to improve posture and, thereby, improve mood and outlook.

The specialty program I have developed helps to change the mindset of depressed people through individualized exercises. This is accomplished by replacing impaired body messages to the mind with more healthy body movements, consistent with those of non-depressed people. Science has shown that mood affects posture, and posture affects mood.

Want to help your patients, literally, *stand up to depression*? You're invited to come spend time with me to learn more about PTM©.

Just contact me at 781.899.6289 or
fairbend@physicaltherapyforthemind.com.

CPSIA information can be obtained
at www.ICGtesting.com
Printed in the USA
LVHW011959181119
637668LV00011BA/401